MW00953641

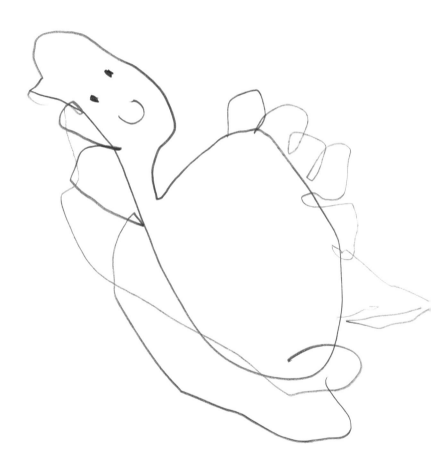

ANGER MANAGEMENT FOR PARENTS RAISING CHILDREN WITH ADHD AND AUTISM

How To Stop Losing Your Temper, Manage Your Emotions, And Build a Better Relationship with Your Special Needs Child

Sharon Daven

© Copyright _____ 2021 - All rights reserved.

The content contained within this book may not be reproduced, duplicated or transmitted without direct written permission from the author or the publisher.

Under no circumstances will any blame or legal responsibility be held against the publisher, or author, for any damages, reparation, or monetary loss due to the information contained within this book. Either directly or indirectly. You are responsible for your own choices, actions, and results.

<u>Legal Notice:</u>

This book is copyright protected. This book is only for personal use. You cannot amend, distribute, sell, use, quote or paraphrase any part, or the content within this book, without the consent of the author or publisher.

Disclaimer Notice:

Please note the information contained within this document is for educational and entertainment purposes only. All effort has been executed to present accurate, up to date, and reliable, complete information. No warranties of any kind are declared or implied. Readers acknowledge that the author is not engaging in the rendering of legal, financial, medical or professional advice. The content within this book has been derived from various sources. Please consult a licensed professional before attempting any techniques outlined in this book.

By reading this document, the reader agrees that under no circumstances is the author responsible for any losses, direct or indirect, which are incurred as a result of the use of the information contained within this document, including, but not limited to, — errors, omissions, or inaccuracies.

Your Free Gift

As a way of saying thanks for your purchase, I'm offering this book *BABY SAFETY TIPS* for **FREE** to my readers.

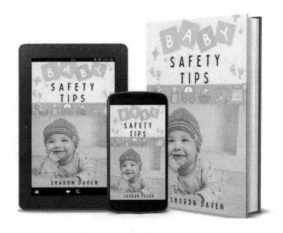

To get instant access **SCAN THE QR CODE:**

Inside this book, you will discover:

- 12-Must have products that will keep your child safe around the home

- Traveling with a baby checklist.

- How to reduce the risk of poisoning in your household.

- Toy Safety Tips.

- Safe bedding practices for infants

If you want to know how to keep your baby safe, make sure to grab this **FREE** book now.

Table of Contents

INTRODUCTION

"Kids don't "make" us yell. They just reveal to us where we have room to grow…"

Shelly Robinson

Is anger a positive or negative feeling? Should expressions of anger be completely thrust out of the home or tolerated to a measure? Is it possible to hit the threshold of stress and just forget to feel anger altogether? These represent the questions that crowd the mind of a mother or father who cares to regulate the home in the greatest degree of love, peace, and happiness.

Research has it that our biological make-up coupled with personal experiences do influence the way we express anger. When we label something as unfair in connection to the overwhelming feelings of powerlessness that may close in on us, five outcomes are usually feasible in the moment.

We could feel threatened, inadequate, vulnerable, victimized, or violated. Yet, regardless of the impact that any of these feelings may render, the hardest drive is toward anger. Is anger bad? You may have a myriad of answers depending on whoever it is you're directing the question.

In delivering honest feedback to your quiz, an overworked employee may flat out tell how an outburst of anger spells doom in creating an avenue of potential job loss. On the other hand, a controlling boss might view anger as the tool for getting things done irrespective of the consequences in breaking out over those under him.

Ask a parent cycling each day on the wheels of various activities and the answers might start to take a different shape. For instance, "anger is inevitable," "anger is normal," or "anger is your priceless armory when dealing with a defiant child." When dealing with a neurodiverse child, a breathtaking answer might not come in handy.

Parents of ADHD or Autistic children probably wind up as the most frustrated especially in situations where they're clueless about their child's condition. Many parents yet to discover the missing pieces in the puzzle of their children's "unusual" attitude might needlessly embark on a dire journey of parenthood while enduring the scalds of stress and regrets that may spring up along the way.

Parents with full-blown knowledge of their child's condition

It is easy to blame anger on unsuspecting parents of ADHD or Autistic children. But let's get real for a second and you will realize that this is beyond a naïve parent thing. Anger is, in fact, every parent thing, showing up in both young and old neurotypical and neurodiverse parents alike.

More than debating who knows what, I think the right way to approach the hot button issue is to dive right into it. My experience of parenting an Autistic child and grand-parenting an ADHD one bears firm witness to both realities. Before I knew about my child's Autistic symptoms, I had bottled up a whole lot of anger that spewed out in the forms of regrets for being a bad mom and resentment toward my baby for not being like his siblings.

And until I uncovered the truth about his situation, I continued to beat myself up and wished he would be 'normal.' Yes, parenting a child without a special condition could turn out as an uphill task. Imagine what handling a continuously hyperactive and super-defiant child will look like. Honestly, each day did feel like opening up a can of trouble without an impression of what you might let loose.

Things quickly changed when I began to acquaint myself with the knowledge of Autism and learned to accept my child for who he really was. Today, I'm a counselor for parents of neurodiverse parents partly because of my desperate quest to find a way around my child's conduct. My interest in enlightening and helping other parents like me navigate the excesses parenting a neurodiverse child may pose has kept me on the path.

More than anything else, I want you to be able to better understand yourself and your child by the time you have finished consuming this material. That would be a box gleefully checked off my bucket list of things I desire this book to accomplish for you. I believe you will also find this book relevant in helping you lose hard knots in particular areas that could hinder an accurate flow with your child.

How ADHD and Autism Impact Your Parenting

Over my five years of counseling parents of neurodiverse children, I have noted that many parents who prioritize finding help for their children are often victims of some unsaid challenges themselves. An unforgettable event which had me unfolding some of these challenges came up on account of a parent who paid me a visit in desperate need of help in dealing with his ADHD child.

While I obtain permission to talk about some of my clients' stories to encourage or educate other parents, I purposely withhold their names and personal details for privacy's sake. Hence the story you're about to read has been stripped of the actual names and the particular details tweaked alongside. But the gist is genuine and you can always glean from it.

Michael was a single dad saddled with the responsibility of caring for his six-year-old since his wife's demise about two years ago. Shortly, he began to notice some signs in his toddler but discarded them while he battled with grieving his late wife. Several months rolled by and the symptoms glared all the more. He decided to see a therapist and I got recommended.

We wasted no time in burrowing into his observations about his child as my diagnosis soon stamped the child as an autistic child. Michael kept returning to me as the months passed and we developed a regimen to help his child perform at optimum capacity. After applying the prepared timetable and allotted medication for close to eighteen months, I was surprised to see Michael waddle into my office to complain about needing help.

This time not his son but he himself required the help. Due to the generous amount of time, effort, and health invested in following his son's special schedule, Michael felt he was falling behind on his usual life. A natural born athlete, his 6ft frame and passion contributed in making him a star at the basketball court which he normally played with friends at 8:30 pm every day.

Since his son's situation, he has cut back on that and many other necessities as he counts them. This seemingly imposed sacrifice he must make for his son to survive in the world is stored up in his system as large doses of bitterness and distress. He narrated that he felt he must have converted those negativities into more negativity as he now relates to his son with anger sometimes. "Maybe there's something you can do to help me…" He begged.

Stigmatization, stress, burn out, and financial issues are vices that may lead to anger when parenting a neurodiverse child. Whether you're suffering from underlying causes of anger as I've listed above or you're in the full-fledged stage of showing anger toward yourself, your spouse, or your child, I have some amazing news for you. Hear me out!

You can still make a 360 degree return to the point where gentle parenting becomes the ultimate. Can I guess I know what you're thinking: "but my child isn't a 'normal' child to adhere to gentle parenting?" To that I say you may have to taste and see to believe that miracles do happen! Friend, you can help your child, reduce your fatigue, and get set to have another child after the current

ADHD or Autistic child, provided you want to. Continue reading this book to expose yourself to the secrets!

What this book holds for you

In *Anger Management for Parents Raising Children with ADHD And Autism,* you're about to

- Learn and understand the various root causes of anger in the journey of parenting your ADHD or Autistic child.

- Develop a lasting solution to fix the bad breaks that interrupt how you cater for your child

- Design a routine that helps you to enjoy the kind of life you desire and deserve as an individual and simultaneously answer to your familial responsibility with little or no stress.

- Initiate a new system that places you on the fast lane of bonding with your child like a parenting pro.

- Acquaint yourself with the diverse styles of anger capable of being displayed, learn how to handle them, explore practical ways to manage and subdue them, and finally assemble the tools required to keep you afloat the flood

of triggers that may come your way.

CHAPTER ONE

ADHD AND AUTISM— DIGGING INTO THE BASICS

"It is not our differences that divide us. It is our inability to

recognize, accept, and celebrate those differences."

-Audre Lorde

Judging from the junk of misconceptions flying about, it is quite expected whenever I get tons of demeaning statements that reveal the different perspectives people have about the subject of neurodiversity. But what holds true? In 1998, an Australian sociologist, Judy Singer, coined the word "neurodiversity" in an attempt to help us recognize that everyone's brain develops in a unique way.

When mentioning neurodiversity, most people tend to think of autism as the only neurodiverse condition that exists, but that is not true. The likes of attention deficit hyperactivity disorder (ADHD), dyslexia, dyscalculia, Down syndrome, and Tourette's syndrome are all categorized under neurodiversity.

According to a 2020 study carried out by Birkbeck University of London, Department of Organizational Psychology: In London and the UK, 15-20 percent of people identify as neurodiverse. An estimated 10% of individuals receive dyslexia diagnosis, 6% receive a dyspraxia diagnosis, 5% receive an ADHD diagnosis, and 1-2% receive an autistic diagnosis.

In contrast to other medical conditions, neurodiversity lacks a recognized treatment. However, there are numerous tactics that can help control the symptoms, as demonstrated by the growing number of testimonies from neurodivergent and parents of children with special needs.

I recall my initial encounter with Katherine. I went to get some cheese and ham at the North Star Mall as I needed to prepare some cheeseburgers for the weekend. Katherine had an enormous smile on her face.

"Hello, Sharon!" She said as she came closer basking with excitement. She told me her friend had bought my book on autism for her the moment she learned about her 7-year-old son—Edward—being diagnosed with the disorder. Edward had struggled with severe emotional irregularities. Katherine narrated how she implemented the relaxation exercise and break-time strategies to help him manage his emotions.

Standing there watching her, I could see the joy that emanated from her heart. I never asked how she could recognize me on a whim but I sure commended her courage in seeking help for her child. Speaking of parenting a neurodiverse child, the flight just took off after you have secured help for your child. Greater work lies in gaining adequate help yourself. I hope this book will be of magnificent help in addressing and managing obvious or subtle anger issues.

Amaya's Transition

Amaya found being a single mother at the youthful age of 19 to be more than enough trouble. Having yet to come to terms with the fact that Marcus, her 24-year-old boyfriend, would rather pursue his dream of becoming an aeronautical engineer than marry her, she is still in shock at how to gather herself and move on with life.

She was forced to accept her new situation when she tested positive for a medical checkup and was taken to the hospital by her older sister Susan, who discovered her after she had passed out that Tuesday morning. Now, ten years later, Mai, her daughter, is in second grade. Mai was still having trouble with her education, even though kids her age were already in grade 4. News from her school never ceased to flow. She was constantly absent-minded during class and engaging with her classmates was never something she found fascinating. It appeared that she was either sitting by herself or painting.

That was all I needed to hear that day when Amaya came into Mia's company into my office. As I immersed myself in the details of Amaya's grievance regarding her daughter, I sent a chic glance Mai's way. By now, Mia was sketching on the blank A4 paper that was resting with other piles of blank A4 papers on my desk. She looked away and out, unbothered by the conversation going on in front of her. And caring little on whether the discourse rallied around her or if it were a mere headline of the daily news, she was lost in her own world.

Amaya was even more devastated to learn that her kid had ADHD. Her brown eyes were displaying her rage. I knew then that I had to give her a different perspective on the matter. I walked over to her agonized seat and gave her a copy of my book, **ADHD Positive Parenting for Boys and Girls**. I was aware of how ignorance affects parents of neurodiverse kids. I wouldn't prefer for her to experience the same setbacks like other parents of neurodiverse kids did.

Few days after the dead of winter, I received a letter—nearly eight months since Amaya visited my office.

Hello, Sharon.

I sincerely appreciate your insightful book on ADHD and your assistance in helping me look past my limitations. I was almost done with Mai when I came to your office that day. I was sick of parenting a child like her, so I decided to send her to my parents as soon as she was diagnosed with ADHD.

But I knew better after reading the masterpiece you provided me. And I'm confident in saying that my Mia has made significant progress—not only academically—after putting all of your suggested strategies into practice.

She just received an award from her school for being the most inventive artist during an art exhibition for students in grades 3 and 4.

Instead of focusing on her limitations, I now acknowledge and appreciate her qualities. My heart goes out to you for caring deeply and making sure I do what is right and not what I feel. I didn't drop the ball in my parenting game because of you.

Warm regards,

Amaya W.

For every neurodiverse child out there, there are ceaseless potentials unlocked within them. You have to come to the point where you view them beyond their underdeveloped brains and start seeing that, though your child was diagnosed with ASD, some of the uncommon strengths that come with ASD individuals are: fine-detail processing memory, honesty, high concentration level, and sensory awareness.

The image below shows the intriguing strengths of different categories of neurodiverse condition.

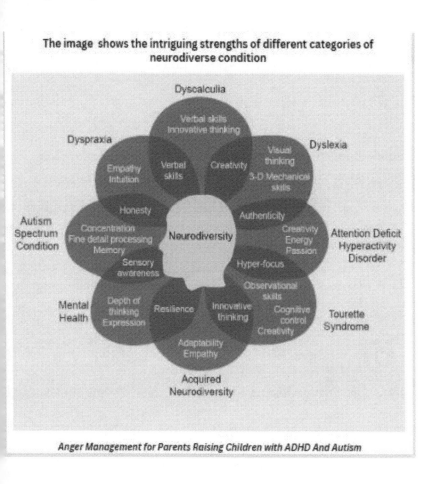

The image shows the intriguing strengths of different categories of neurodiverse condition

Anger Management for Parents Raising Children with ADHD And Autism

Recognizing Individual Differences

Knowing not to ignore one child in favor of the other or compare their neurodiverse child to the neurotypical ones sounds counterintuitive to the majority of parents who have only one neurodiverse child among other kids. The temptation to rate them all using the same method is constant. What benefit, though, can this have? Not good. Rather, the notion that they are not good enough ultimately wins them over.

Lucia's Superpowers

It wasn't until two years ago that Jack realized his daughter Lucia, 16, suffered from a comorbid disorder that combines ASD and ADHD. He now realizes the peculiarities that have shaped Lucia into the person she is. As he thinks back on their past miscommunications, how she suddenly got angry with everyone, why she frequently disobeyed his orders, and why she constantly complained about not wanting to go out with her high school classmates even though they won't stop hanging around the house.

She occasionally experienced autistic meltdowns but was unaware of them. Everyone believed she was being foolish. Yet, one bit of discovery and the story seem different now. Jack says that knowing Lucia has autism made it easier for him to accept her abilities and recognize some of her limits.

For Jack, it was always her creative intellect. As someone with hyperactive ADHD, she is known for her hyper-focus when doing what she is passionate about, so it was only natural for her to spot issues and come up with answers in her thoughts before anyone even asked. His mind began to race with the following question: "How do I help my girl light up her potential?"

First of all, he urged her to enroll in Oklahoma City University's project management classes. In addition, she applied for internships at companies that needed her particular set of abilities. Given that one of the potential consequences of ADHD is poor time management, he also provided her with an action priority matrix to aid in her time management. Realizing that she occasionally has trouble finishing things, it was also part of the idea to divide the activities into smaller chunks particularly when it becomes too much.

Rather than engaging in their customary comparison-gaming, Lucia began to believe that she possessed the necessary skills to excel in her own domain. Probably, you wish that all parents could be like Jack. I also hoped for that. But with Andy, the scripts were different.

Andy's dilemma

It was summertime off. My daughter would never pass up the chance to spend the holidays with my 5-year-old grandson at San Antonio, as usual. My last son, Peter, usually had his best moments during this period. It was his chance to have a playmate and younger brother nearby.

After we'd finished watching the American TV family series The Waltons, my grandson asked me a question that made me shiver. "Grandma, is it possible for someone to hate a child she gave birth to?" What? From where was this coming? I asked him what was wrong and who told him about hating someone.

It seemed like he noticed the stunned silence on my face right away. "No, grand, Andy told me that his family doesn't like him," he answered, bowing his head. Whoa! Andy, who is this? I inquired without pausing to let him catch his breath.

Apparently, Andy, a classmate, has an ADHD diagnosis as well. My kid had always noticed that Andy always had a dejected expression on his face whenever the closing bell rings and would prefer being in school than going home unlike other kids, based on what I was told. This prompted him to enquire as to what was wrong, and it was then that he discovered his mother always separates him from his siblings. One would think that since he is the last child, they would spoil him, but apparently the opposite is true.

She believes that his escape from rebellion comes from the melting of punishments. Sadly, Andy never gets to meet the expectations his mother has set for her children. It is clear that she had high standards. His mom had adopted a policy of reprimanding, comparing, and punishing instead of helping him manage the disorder.

My grandson's tears were almost visible to me. It was at that moment that I realized that many parents of neurodivergent children are still fighting ignorance. If you don't know what makes your special-needs child different, you'll inevitably talk them out of your life and cause them to become distant.

Impact on parenting dynamics

Many people consider parenting to be among the most difficult tasks to complete. How come? You may ask. I can tell you as someone who has been married for more than 20 years. Before we had children, my husband and I had plans and structures set out for our ideal home. It was our intention to teach our children parenting skills that would allow them to approach us freely and express their opinions without fear of our disapproval. However, we learned not to make tweaks after we had our autistic son, Peter. Now, I want you to know what parenting strategies to use at your house. How can this dynamic support your child who has neurodiversity?

A study conducted in 2015 by Baumrind contributed to the deciphering of the various parental dynamic's issues. It includes the many approaches parents take to raising their kids. The methods and frameworks used in parenting.

Different Styles of Parenting

1. Authoritarian parenting: Remember Andy? Yes, I guess. His mother raised him according to this model. This is setting up high expectations for your kids' behavior without allowing them to fully see the rationale behind them. When it comes to disobedience, this parenting style seems to always resort to punishment.

2. Permissive parenting: The capacity to treat their kids like friends is one aspect of this parenting approach that really sticks out. Punishments for misbehavior are applied infrequently.

3. Authoritative parenting: This happens to be my favorite. It gives room for Interactive conversation between your kids and you. With this style of parenting the kids tend to know the reason behind the policies and standards you set for them as parents.

How does your parenting styles affect your neurodivergent child and vice versa

"The consequences of every act are included in the act itself," as said by George Orwell, best describes this situation. Regardless of the parenting style you select, outcomes will inevitably follow. Rather, the better thing to ask is: will it be a good or bad one? Rigid parenting has the potential to impact your children in the following ways:

1. **Increased anxiety**: An authoritarian parenting strategy could backfire since neurodivergent have trouble in strict surroundings.
2. It diminishes their sense of self.
3. It builds a barrier between you and your child.

As parents:

1. **Anger**: This is the primary effect of neurodiversity on parenting. Just like the story of Olivia I shared earlier, a lot of parents get angry with the fact that they have to be

the ones raising a neurodiverse child. They see it as a limitation and a failure. Limitations because being a parent of a neurodivergent child may not permit you to participate in certain activities, like frequent outings, especially for those with autistic kids who sometimes act differently in public.

2. **Frustration**: The thought that your kids aren't meeting up to the standard you've set for them is enough of a reason to be down for most parents.

The right perspective on parenting

As I attempt to wrap up this chapter, let me note that if you genuinely want to parent your neurodivergent child more effectively, you must adopt the appropriate mindset. It will be safer for you to consciously use the following strategies when raising your special-needs child if you know how you should see them and how your preferred parenting approach can make matters worse for both of you and them:

1. Honor their abilities.

2. Take up their cause.

3. Enable them to reach their greatest potential, just like Jack did.

I'll go over the connection between anger, stress, and parenting in the upcoming chapter. Thus, helping you recognize the reasons behind your emotions and learn how to identify the things that make you angry, as well as early warning signals and coping techniques. It's certain that this will be a shift for you.

TAKE HOME:

- Every neurodivergent child has embedded in them ceaseless potentials that requires you to help them tap from it.

- Nothing can change beyond your perception. This is true for neurodiversity.

- Your child's condition can impact on the dynamics of your parenting. Hence, first know your child then proceed to know you can best come in.

CHAPTER TWO

THE LINK BETWEEN

PARENTING, STRESS AND

ANGER

"Between stimulus and response, there is a space. In that space

is our power to choose our response."

-Viktor Frankl

In the previous chapter, you were enlightened on ADHD and autism neurodiversity. You got to understand how to view a child with ADHD and Autism. On a closer view you discover that each child has individual differences and know that different ADHD or Autistic children have different characteristics, and no two ADHD or Autistic children are the same. Along the line, you got insights on how ADHD and Autism impacts the parenting dynamics. And you finally familiarized yourself with the right way and perspective of parenting such a child.

Welcome to a pivotal chapter delving into the intricate link between parenting, stress, and anger. Here, I embark on a journey of self-discovery, unraveling the layers that contribute to the complex emotions parents often grapple with. I'll navigate the landscape of why you feel the way you do, exploring triggers unique to the parental experience.

In the first section, our focus turns inward as I embark on the crucial task of identifying personal triggers for anger. Understanding these triggers becomes the compass guiding your journey toward more mindful parenting. As I delve deeper, I'll shed light on recognizing early signs of anger. Through introspection and keen self-awareness, you empower yourself to intercept and navigate these emotions before they escalate.

Friend, I understand how the feeling of parenting may be very much overwhelming at times. I'm acquainted with those moments where frustration brews, and the unexpected catch you off guard. Parenthood isn't a pristine journey but a messy, beautiful mosaic of highs and lows. I know there's always a struggle of balancing your needs with the relentless demands of caring for your children.

A parent in a cape

This calls to mind an episode while growing up. My Mother would always buy gorgeous clothes and shoes for my siblings and I from time to time when we ask for it or sometimes when we don't even ask for it. One day I just sat down and started wondering when my mother got something really nice for herself, and trust me it was really a long time ago. So, I summoned the courage to ask her why she's always buying things for us her children without even getting one for herself and she said "You are my future, I need to take care of you before myself, I wouldn't want my past to be better than my future, you know."

Indeed, there are times when self-care feels like a distant luxury. The relentless cycle of daily tasks often leaves you wondering, "Should I prioritize myself or my kids first?" I am here to explore with you that dilemma, recognizing the internal tug-of-war that every parent endures.

In the intricate dance of parenthood, I want to pause in the quiet rhythm and acknowledge the extraordinary risks you take every day for the well-being of your children. It's not just about the sleepless nights, the sacrifices, or the constant juggling act — it's about the profound courage it takes to be a parent.

I understand the weight you carry, the worries that linger in the quiet hours, and the decisions that shape your child's world. The risks you take aren't always visible, but they're felt in the quiet moments of uncertainty and the loud moments of unconditional love.

From the moment you welcomed your child into your arms, you embarked on a journey of vulnerability. Every decision, every sacrifice, and every moment of worry is a testament to your unwavering dedication. The risks you willingly take are not just part of parenting; they're a profound expression of your love and commitment.

So, here's to you — the risk-takers, the dream-weavers, the everyday heroes. In the grand tapestry of parenting, your courage stands as a beacon. I see you; I acknowledge you, and I stand beside you in awe of the risks you take for the ones you love the most.

Identifying Personal Triggers for Anger

Meet Sarah, a dedicated mother to Alex, a young boy with autism. Their daily life, though rich with love, carries its own set of challenges. One evening, as they engaged in a seemingly ordinary routine of homework, an unexpected challenge arose. The task, which most would view as straightforward, became a minefield of frustration for Alex. The atmosphere in the room shifted, setting the stage for a testing moment.

In the midst of what appeared to be a simple homework session, frustration mounted for both Alex and Sarah. The unfolding scene was not merely about the academic task; it became a reflection of the broader challenges they faced. As the tension escalated, Sarah felt a familiar knot tightening within her — a blend of frustration, helplessness, and a tinge of guilt.

In the aftermath of the homework meltdown, Sarah took a moment to reflect. What was it about these situations that consistently triggered such a visceral response? Through introspection, she discovered that it wasn't just about the immediate challenge; it was a culmination of the broader struggles they faced daily. The trigger, it seemed, was rooted in the feeling of inadequacy as a parent and the societal pressure to conform to conventional norms.

Sarah's story unveils a common trigger for parents of autistic children — the unspoken societal expectations that often cast a shadow on their unique parenting journey. The pressure to conform to conventional norms, especially in situations like homework, became a silent trigger for Sarah's anger.

Armed with this newfound awareness, Sarah embarked on a journey of understanding. Rather than viewing the triggers as weaknesses, she recognized them as invitations for growth. Each trigger became a signpost, guiding her toward a deeper comprehension of her own emotions and the intricate dynamics of parenting an autistic child.

Sarah's story reflects the power of identifying personal triggers for anger as a parent. It's not just about addressing the surface-level challenges but delving into the deeper currents that shape our emotional responses. By embracing self-reflection, parents can navigate these triggers with a newfound resilience and foster an environment of understanding for both themselves and their children.

In the vast canvas of parenting, recognizing personal triggers is not a sign of weakness but a courageous step toward creating a more empathetic and harmonious family dynamic.

Recognizing Early Signs of Anger

While navigating the unique path of raising an autistic child, recognizing the early signs of anger becomes a pivotal tool. Let's explore this imperative aspect through the lens of a parent, Mark, as he discerns the subtle indicators of brewing anger within.

Mark is a devout father to Lily—an effervescent child on the autism spectrum. Their days, filled with triumphs and trials, hold moments of unpredictability. One evening, during a family outing to a bustling fair, Lily's sensory overload reached a climax, setting the stage for a potential challenge.

Amidst the vibrant fairgrounds, Lily's sensory response to the bustling environment intensified. Her distress manifested in subtle cues – increased stimming, fleeting eye contact, and a heightened restlessness. These early signs, imperceptible to many, were the gentle whispers of a potential storm brewing within Lily.

As Lily's distress escalated, Mark recognized the signs of impending overwhelm. It wasn't just about the external stimuli; it was a delicate dance between understanding Lily's needs and preempting a potential meltdown.

Armed with this newfound awareness, Mark embraced a proactive approach. Rather than waiting for a full-blown meltdown, he intervened early. He sought to create a calm, supportive environment for Lily, preempting the escalation of her distress.

Recognizing the early signs of anger or distress in parenting an autistic child is akin to deciphering a gentle language – it's not always explicit but requires attentive listening. By tuning into these subtle cues, parents can proactively navigate challenging moments, fostering an environment of understanding and support for their children.

Developing Coping Strategies

In the vibrant tapestry of social gatherings, Emma found herself embarking on a unique journey as a mother to Ethan, a spirited child on the autism spectrum. Amid the laughter and chatter of a community event, an unexpected twist awaited, etching a chapter of resilience and growth.

It was a bustling community event, filled with laughter and the hum of conversations. Ethan, an imaginative soul with an affinity for routines, encountered a disruption that sent ripples through the carefully orchestrated social dance. In the midst of the lively gathering, the unexpected clash of colors became the trigger for a storm of emotions.

Emma, threading the needle of daily challenges, felt the stirrings of anger. It wasn't aimed at Ethan; it was a response to the unexpected disruption in their well-rehearsed routine. The vibrant chaos unfolding in Ethan's interactions mirrored the internal uproar within Emma.

As Ethan's distress heightened, Emma's initial composure waned. In this whirlwind of frustration, her anger, laced with the weight of societal expectations, emerged. The lively social gathering echoed with clashing emotions — the vibrant chaos mirrored the internal commotion of both mother and son.

In this increase of emotions, Emma questioned the fairness of their journey. The weight of being an advocate, a caregiver, and a source of unwavering support pressed down. The storm reached its zenith, demanding a decision from Emma — to succumb to the anger or to channel it into understanding. In this pivotal moment, Emma chose love over the tumult of emotions. Amidst the lively gathering, she embraced a moment of clarity, realizing that the anger wasn't a betrayal but a plea for understanding.

In the aftermath, Emma embarked on a journey of enlightenment. Fueled by determination, she delved into research about autism, seeking to comprehend Ethan's world more deeply. Simultaneously, Emma, recognizing the toll on her mental well-being, sought solace in therapy. It wasn't just for her; it was an investment in becoming the steadfast advocate Ethan needed.

Emma's story unfolded not just amidst a social gathering but in the heart of a community. Her anger, a natural response to the challenges, became the catalyst for positive change. Emma transformed it into a force for understanding, advocacy, and a deeper connection with Ethan.

In the complex and beautiful journey of parenting an autistic child, the ability to recognize early signs of anger emerges as a profound skill. Through the lens of parents like Mark, who navigate the nuanced landscape with resilience and attentiveness, you discover that these early signals are more than just precursors to potential challenges—they are opportunities for proactive intervention, understanding, and growth.

By acknowledging the subtle cues, parents can transform potential moments of distress into stepping stones toward harmonious parenting. It's a dance of empathy, where the parent becomes attuned to the unique language of their child's emotions. The story of recognizing these early signs isn't just about averting meltdowns; it's about fostering an environment where each family member can thrive.

In this concluding note, I celebrate the parents who, with love and awareness, navigate the intricate dynamics of parenting an autistic child. Through early recognition, they paint a canvas of understanding, turning potential storms into moments of connection and growth. May every early sign be met with compassion, turning the journey into a symphony of harmony and resilience.

Chapter 3 will take you through the process of collaborating with professionals to understand individual parenting styles for children with ADHD and autism.

TAKE HOME:

- The ability to recognize early signs of distress or anger in an autistic child is a powerful tool for parents.

- The subtle cues exhibited by an autistic child, such as changes in behavior or sensory responses, convey a nuanced language that parents can learn to interpret.

- Parents who engage in self-reflection, like Mark in the discussed scenario, gain a deeper understanding of their own triggers and emotional responses.

- The journey of parenting an autistic child is filled with challenges, but through early recognition and understanding, these challenges can be transformed into opportunities for connection and growth.

- Achieving harmony in the parenting journey involves not only recognizing early signs but also responding with empathy and constructive action.

CHAPTER THREE

COLLABORATING AND STRATEGIZING

"The purpose of therapy is not to remove suffering but to move through it to an enlarged consciousness that can sustain the polarity of painful opposites."

- James Hollis

I hope that the last chapter helped you to work through the early signs of anger and the different coping strategies to achieve a smooth parenting journey. This was accomplished by helping you understand why you feel the way you do and the triggers responsible for that resentment you may feel towards parenting your neurodivergent child.

This chapter is intended to assist you in comprehending the role of outside assistance in positioning you for a better experience as a parent. You will learn how to use different tactics, tools, and strategies necessary to support you along the way. Also, you'll have access to the resources you need to talk strategically with your child so that your messages are understood and their needs are met.

Collaborating with professional

When raising a child with special needs, you're probably going to feel overwhelmed especially if you approach it with no stated plan. How do I know this? I felt the same way at first while raising my Peter—my autistic child. Particularly when there were no resources available to serve as guardians and I had to begin learning from my own experience.

Of course, considering the opinions of other people in raising my child was the last thing I wanted to do. But when it felt like I was going through hell and had no alternatives but to keep on going, I fell back. I began my fierce search for answers, for ease, for solution of some sort. I found answers after delving into an ocean of research work and went on to become a professional myself because of this same reason. I must tell you though that while my profession may have prospered by self-effort, my personal comfort and timely courage only soared on the wings of actual consultation with other experts.

Below I have presented relevant strategies constituent of the advice I gleaned sitting through sessions of therapy and pre-planned groups. I expect that you'll surf through the multiple options discussed and stick to the various ones that might work for you. Without further ado, let's look at these named strategies experts suggest beginning with the best strategies to help you schedule a session with one.

Seeking answers for Peter

I believed I could handle everything on my own after devoting nearly eight hours of thorough work that evening to researching Peter's case and potential answers for his disturbing reality. Since these were the main areas we were struggling with, I decided to start by doing more in-depth study on how to help a child listen to commands and develop the habit of finishing chores.

He frequently became overwhelmed by large activities, so I came across websites that discussed reducing those seemingly massive tasks down for them and minimizing distractions around work areas—homework tables. I put my findings into practice right away. A testimony of a twenty-five-year-old American entrepreneur named Greg acted as my guide. Greg had previously disclosed that he was diagnosed at the age of twenty while working as a media consultant for a US transformation firm at the time. On a mission to incapacitate the grip of the ADHD weakness on him, he got into the habit of breaking down large jobs which spiraled up his ability to finish them.

Summer vacation was around the corner of that year. So, I looked for a less distracting spot at home in preparation for his schoolwork and other projects. It ought to be a tranquil space where he could unwind, process his feelings, find some peace, and just disconnect from the outside world. We had a prayer corner which everyone knows is for quiet and calm reflection away from the every-day boisterous schedule. I decided to expand its use as Peter's safe spot.

I installed a task manager app on his iPad so he could get notified periodically 10 minutes to his next task. I made sure to follow

Greg's testimony willy-nilly but things didn't change as much. No doubt, Peter improved in his ability to complete tasks but not in his ability to socialize, stay calm, respond to orders nor with his ability to remain on cue after being interrupted.

What was I not doing right? I was getting frustrated. Just then the thought of speaking with Joanne — a family friend came to mind. I put a call across to Joanne and pour out my frustrations. That's when she brought up the necessity of getting expert assistance. "Sharon, although I can't claim to fully understand how you're feeling, I can tell you that right now what you need is a shoulder to cry on."

With these words, she shared Dr. Francis' contact with me. He served as a psychiatrist consultant for individuals having attention deficit hyperactivity disorder. Joanne said she was confident he could assist. I let out a long breath when I heard those words.

For both my son Peter and me, this marked the beginning of a major transition. I was naively following Greg's testimony, forgetting that no two neurodiverse are the same. And until we met with Dr. Francis the following week did, I realize that Peter might have Autism rather than ADHD. It was then that he opened my eyes to the lapses I had never seen. Then it hit me that even when my instincts proposed Peter could be autistic, I blindly subscribed to Greg's words without stopping to check.

Working With Therapists and Counselors

Building a relationship with your therapist is essential when working with them. It's crucial to remember that not every counselor will be the ideal match for you and your kid. It is for this reason that you must look around for a counselor who best fits you. When Peter and I drove from San Antonio to San Marcos to see Dr. Francis, this was my first prayer. In order for me to determine whether or not we would like to continue the session with the psychiatric specialist, he provided us with a free 15-minute consultation.

When we saw Dr. Francis for the first time, the fifty-year-old American man with the skimmed-look greeted us with a smile that said, "I've been expecting you." Sharon, good day. He sat us down and gave me an ADHD clinical questionnaire, stating that he needed the answers to help guide our sessions.

We had a two-hour session. However, since I started raising Peter, these two hours have been the finest of my life. I was able to access the session's depth by following the simple guidelines provided. You could wonder what these instructions are, and I've assisted you in classifying them.

1. **Refrain from masking the circumstances**: Not until I began receiving counseling services a few years ago did I truly get this lesson. In therapy, some parents may be too traumatized, ashamed, or embarrassed for a variety of reasons to express their deepest fears and feelings. Be free. In order to help you, the therapist requires your assistance.

2. **Recognize that therapy is a team effort:** Laura Mueller, a certified independent clinical social worker, clarifies in her advice. "The most effective therapy strikes a balance between assisting the client and letting them come to their

own conclusions." You cannot expect the finest outcomes by relying solely on your therapist to complete the work. You also play a part.

3. **Know that your homework assignments are an extension of your therapy sessions**: The minute-by-minute assignments Dr. Francis gave me back then was one of the things I liked. One of them required me to mark an achievement calendar. This calendar aids in keeping track of how frequently I celebrate my son on his small wins. You may give him presents, take him on a tour, or simply give him permission to spend an additional hour doing what he enjoys.

Joining Support Groups

An autism or ADHD support group is a community of people who get together to share stories, offer encouragement, and educate one another on what it's like to live with autism or ADHD. The group may consist of loved ones, family members, and those with autism or ADHD. They may also comprise experts with an interest in ADHD and how it affects day-to-day functioning.

If Dr. Francis stressed anything during our sessions, it's that a support group is not a substitute for a therapist or doctor. It serves only as a complement. A support group can, nevertheless, provide you with certain benefits.

1. **The knowledge that you are not alone:** This frequently helps people who are struggling with stigma. You will meet a great deal of people in the support group who are going through similar struggles as you, whether they are recently diagnosed or have achieved success with their therapy or medication.

2. **Enhances self-awareness and social abilities:** It is beneficial and good for members to meet and converse with one another. This can assist in overcoming the social disengagement and isolation that the illness frequently causes.

3. **Access to real-life- practically helpful information:** As people in the group share their stories, they tend to offer

practical tips, resources, and strategies for addressing their diagnosed issues and progressing in their recovery. Groups may focus on educating their members about coping skills and putting them into practice.

4. **It gives you the opportunity to help others:** As you benefit from the group experience, you are also able to help others grow and make progress by sharing with positivity and care.

Connecting With School Resources

There are two ways to meet your child's teacher to address your child's condition. The first way is to inform your child's teacher about the reality of your child's neurodiverse condition. I emphasized that in one of my previous titled ADHD Positive Parenting for Boys and Girls. Working with the school to create a conducive learning environment for your child is an immense way to get the school invested in effectively training your child.

Conversely, you can meet with your child's teacher to find out about your child's improvements. It's a way of getting attune with how an improvement in school inversely leads to advancement at home. To obtain and maximize this kind of feedback requires an intentional approach that'll enable the instructor to deliver beneficial comments.

1. ***Meet at intervals***- It is crucial to make your child's teacher aware of your child's condition early enough before or at the beginning of the school year. Getting information that will enhance the relationship between you and your child calls for intermittent meetings during the school year.

   This method involves setting up a system which positions your child's teacher as your partner in your child's education team. You let them know of the newest changes your family might be undergoing and how that may impact your child's education. Or ask for their hearts on how to row through situations that may pose a storm to your child's education.

2. ***Encourage backtracking***- Asking your child's instructor to contact you during any significant case will ensure that

the communication lines are open. As such, it is easier for you to access remarkable details about your child's behavior in the swiftness of time.

Your child's instructor will be able to give a heads up in time regarding the situation where there's a decline or spike in behavior and you can leverage the received updates in moderating how you relate to your child. Doing this will assist you to regulate your actions in line with the latest happenings in your child's life.

3. *Establish Parent-Groups*- Joint "suffering" breeds unity. Linking up with other parents who are encountering similar conditions in their children would go a long way to help you assess your child's behavior. The truth is, some parents have more experience than the others owing to the number of years they've dealt with their neurodiverse children. Stories from their standpoint will certainly offer a way to solve health, social, or mental puzzles around your child's condition.

Compelling your child's tutor to connect you with willing parents would help you in forming solid friendships or partnerships with treasurable and lasting bonds.

Engaging the right strategies

Now that we've established the fact that there's a need to collaborate with others in parenting your special-needs child, it's also important that you understand that it is your sole responsibility to engage the strategies you learn in your parenting journey. This is where the magic lies. In the next few paragraphs, I'll be showing how you can rightly engage the strategies, starting with your parenting styles, then your communication patterns, and setting expectations for your special-needs child.

Parenting styles and strategies

In the first chapter, I discussed the three primary styles of parenting as outlined by Diane Baumrind. I briefly discussed authoritarian, authoritative, and permissive ideas. Let's examine these parenting methods and the appropriate tactics they employ in more detail.

The picture below displays the many approaches of parenting.

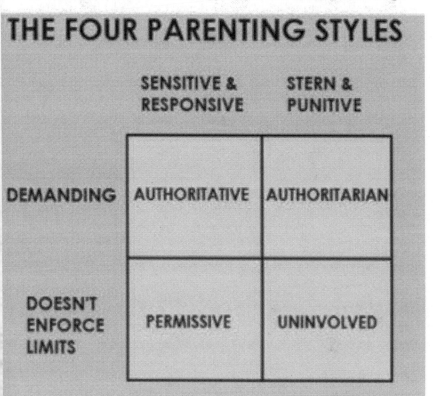

This image shows the many approaches of parenting.

THE FOUR PARENTING STYLES

	SENSITIVE & RESPONSIVE	STERN & PUNITIVE
DEMANDING	AUTHORITATIVE	AUTHORITARIAN
DOESN'T ENFORCE LIMITS	PERMISSIVE	UNINVOLVED

Anger Management for Parents Raising Children with ADHD And Autism

Researchers McCoby and Martin (1983) added the fourth parenting style category: uninvolved parenting style. In that they don't uphold rules, absentee parents are similar to permissive parents. However, detached parents lack the warmth and nurturing of permissive parents. They gave food and shelter to children, but not much more.

Additionally, Diane Baumrind's was restated. Two classifications of parenting styles were established by them: responsiveness and self-regulation. The former refers to the degree to which parents consciously cultivate individuality, self-control, and self-assertion by being aware of, accommodating, and compliant with their children's unique needs and expectations. Baumrind (1991) describes "the claims parents make on children to become integrated into the family whole, by their maturity demands, supervision, disciplinary efforts, and willingness to confront the child who disobeys" as being both non-demanding and demanding less.

Let's examine the different strategies these parenting styles use in the picture below.

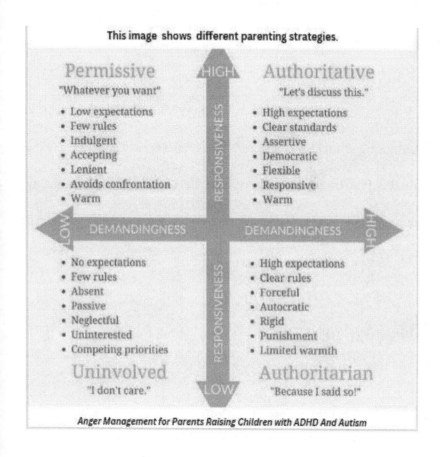

This image shows different parenting strategies.

Permissive
"Whatever you want"
- Low expectations
- Few rules
- Indulgent
- Accepting
- Lenient
- Avoids confrontation
- Warm

Authoritative
"Let's discuss this."
- High expectations
- Clear standards
- Assertive
- Democratic
- Flexible
- Responsive
- Warm

HIGH RESPONSIVENESS

LOW DEMANDINGNESS — HIGH DEMANDINGNESS

LOW RESPONSIVENESS

- No expectations
- Few rules
- Absent
- Passive
- Neglectful
- Uninterested
- Competing priorities

- High expectations
- Clear rules
- Forceful
- Autocratic
- Rigid
- Punishment
- Limited warmth

Uninvolved
"I don't care."

Authoritarian
"Because I said so!"

Anger Management for Parents Raising Children with ADHD And Autism

I'm aware that you might have other kids who aren't neurodivergent, and it wouldn't be a good idea to apply the same pattern for all of them because their needs will undoubtedly differ. This is what personalized parenting aims to achieve.

Personalized parenting, another name for individualized parenting, is just providing for the individual needs of each of your children. It does, however, need that parents watch, get to know their kids very well, and figure out what makes them tick.

With minor adjustments, researchers claim that authoritative parenting is ideal for children who are neurodiverse. This is due to the fact that authoritative parents establish boundaries and expectations with clarity and are kind, caring, and attentive to their children's needs. Why is this?

This kind of parenting involves providing emotional support, constancy, and constructive criticism.

- **Consistency:** Children with ADHD can better understand expectations when there are clear rules and routines in place.

- **Positive reinforcement:** Rewarding excellent behavior with praise and treats helps children stay on course.

- **Emotional support:** A strong parent-child link is created via empathy and understanding, which promotes cooperation and trust.

Communication strategies

How do you pass your message across to your special needs child without making an attempt to affect their well-being? Clear, concise, concrete, and accurate communication is necessary. This is why engaging the following communication strategies is highly recommended.

Keep in mind that, according to the structure of their brains, they find stressful activities that call for a lot of mental effort or even inventiveness, and they quickly lose interest in tasks that don't appeal to them. This includes following your directions. For this reason, I strongly advise parents to refrain from using abstract or airy language while attempting to communicate with their ADHD child as doing so will likely cause them to become frustrated. Instead, use language that is compatible with the ADHD brain.

Use clear, concise, and concrete language whenever possible. For instance, you could state, "Failing to read for an exam makes one fail," rather than "Preparation for an exam increases the risk of low grades." Do you get it? Despite the fact that both statements convey the same idea, the latter is shorter and more direct than the former.

Setting realistic expectations

In 2021 I met with a lady who asked me that, if I claim that Neurodiversity is not a hopeless case, why then can't a neurodivergent do what every other child does. Trust me when I tell you that even a neurotypical child won't act exactly the same way another person's neurotypical child will act. Comparing your ADHD child to the other children is one of the biggest mistakes parents with ADHD children make. The root of the frustration and stress many of these parents encounter even as they attempt to raise their ADHD child is the expectation that these kids would live up to the standard of other kids in terms of academic performance, social development, and other areas. This is why I want you to debunk this misconception and ease your stress.

First of all, you must realize that your ADHD child is different from your other children, and as a result, it is best for you to make a different track for tracking their overall growth. Don't set them up for failure by setting lofty standards. It could be difficult to appreciate their small victories or advancements until you are aware of this truth.

Not only will your child make more progress as a result, but you'll feel less stressed. Be aware that having expectations as a parent is perfectly OK as long as they are directed towards assisting your child in progressing from where they are currently. Get down on their level.

In the next chapter I will describe how to foster self-care as a parent of a neurodiversity. With this knowledge you will learn the importance of self-care, practical strategies to foster self-care and the place of balancing your parental responsibilities.

TAKE HOME:

- Therapy is a team work that requires you to collaborate with professionals for your desired results.

- It is your ability to effectively engage the strategies learned during the collaboration stage that determines what outcome you get

- Your goal while communicating with your neurodiverse child should not be centered on your points being made alone and put into consideration his or her well-being.

CHAPTER FOUR

FOOSTERING SELF-CARE FOR PARENTS

"Almost everything will work again if you unplug it for a few

minutes, including you."

-Anne Lamott

I'm confident that you've already gleaned a great deal of knowledge from the previous chapter. The gems of knowledge you've garnered about working with experts including using the best techniques for your child with special needs will help you as you navigate parenting a neurodivergent child.

In this chapter, I'll be guiding you through the process of regaining your life back and living to the fullest even as you cater for your neurodivergent child. And this is not restricted to whether you're a young mom or dad or a grandparent acclimatizing yourself with your empty-nester years.

In a few moments, you'll figure out why you deserve some attention as well. No doubt, your child needs optimum attention level to blossom in their condition. Yet sacrificing care for yourself on the altar of service to your child is no way to live. To thrive, some necessities cannot be overridden. And to be a parent or guardian who makes a mark in the lives of their child while leaving a mark in the world speaks of dedication to oneself as others come after.

Yes, I dare that you read that well. A vital reason why many parents, especially career women often put a full stop on childbearing after an event of birthing a neurodiverse child rest on a singular reason. They're pressed for time.

You may overlook my words about considering yourself before others but I'm sure you can't shake off your contempt for loss of personal freedom. Caregivers in many foster homes attest to the fact that many ambitious parents whose neurodiverse child takes first place in their childbearing voyage have gone ahead to abandon their children without turning back. I believe the primal reason for this is they think raising an "abnormal" child would circumvent their plans and bring their plans to a standstill. Could this really be the case?

It Begins with You

To make a crude guess: every parent craves a happy time at home with their spouse and children. As a parent, you want to see your children through the different seasons until they're mature enough to live on their own terms. At the same time, you'll give anything to secure their future without making mistakes.

Taking a step back to survey the reality that accompanies upbringing a neurodiverse child may not entirely promise that lifestyle. Looking through the lenses of your child's condition as a disability that warrants you *killing* yourself to satisfy an impeccable growth process would rid you of every courage.

On the flip side, viewing your child's growth, happiness, and stability as an overflow of your own character would give that power boost you need to take charge of your home, career, and life generally. So, apart from the notorious sacrifice you may have erroneously adapted as a way to care for your neurodiverse child, is there another way out to the perfect destination you envisioned?

Maybe. Science has it that human beings behave based on a 2-System decision. System 1 covers the emotional and automatic part of the brain. System 2 is described as the slow and deliberate part responsible for analysis. These two systems interweave and interact together to help us define our behaviors.

According to this study, certain stimuli can improve or limit one's impact on decision making. For instance, going through the motions of mental and physical exhaustion, extremely taxing tasks or time pressure can shut down a person's System 2 thinking making them to solely rely on System 1 judgments.

I'm sure you'll agree with me that if you first of all put yourself in the position where accurate thinking is possible, you'll see a way through the walls. But how do you do that when you're smothered under the heat of increasing obligations and responsibilities that never run out? Well, if you see yourself in the mirror of this experience, then this chapter has been designed for you to offer a lasting solution.

My Encounters

I didn't have it all figured out initially while battling to help my autistic son, Peter. Back then, you would rarely see me mapping out time for myself in the universe of endless duties that typify caring for a neurodiverse kid. I hardly took naps, hardly had time-outs, hardly enjoyed life with my husband and our other children. Bent on helping Peter live the normal life while secretly hoping he'd just be normal in some form, way or shape; I neglected the fact that I was beginning to act as the neurodiverse one.

Always on the go and shifting gears from activity to another left me on a constant level of stress and burnouts. Little things easily infuriated me, I clenched my fists, grinded my teeth, and felt suffocated rapidly gasping for air. This slipped out of hands and my colleague suggested I see a therapist for the fear that I might also be suffering from neurodiversity, even though I had no previous history of depression or insomnia. It took me sometime but I had to take the trip to Dr. Francis's office and circled back to embrace what made the difference—self-care.

Practical Self-Care Strategies

"To be a good parent, you need to take care of yourself so that you can have the physical and emotional energy to take care of your family," says Michelle Obama, an American attorney who served as the country's First Lady. Let's examine some strategies for self-care when raising a child with neurodiversity.

1. Tune In to Your Feelings

"The attempt to escape from pain creates more pain"

-Gabor Mate

You will scarcely find a solution if you're yet to find a problem. I need to repeat at this point in time that you're not a loser for feeling weak. This quote I heard from an anonymous speaker changed my life the very day it came to me. It says: if you feel pain in your body that means there's something wrong with your body and if you feel pain emotionally that means there's something wrong with your mind.

Those words have since then been carved on the canvas of my heart where I call it to memory every time fear coils around my heart like a python. The fear of looking weak and not being enough to handle my life and home, the fear of what people would say if I become vulnerable enough to let them see me crumble. I'll say it's a miracle today that I feel safe to divulge all of my darkest secrets as I counsel other parents both on stage and on paper.

When you start to notice some amount of discomfort and your life starts to generate unwanted heat that sends you sweating in your pants, then it's time to reassess. Pay laser-focused attention to where something feels wrong in your body or mental health. Take the time to get compassionate with yourself as you unclutter the layers that have built up in the past.

Napoleon Hill is popular for his energetic opinion that "Every adversity, every failure, every heartache carries with it the seed of an equal or greater benefit." The pain you feel brings with it a potential for fixture. You can fix it once you can recognize the problem.

2. Feeling Pain in Your Body? – Do this

Maintain Your Body Fuel Level

We talked about the link between Parenting and stress in Chapter 2 of this book and I'll encourage you to refer to it if you need to. According to research, parents of children with autism and ADHD typically have higher cortisol levels—also referred to as the 'stress hormone.' It is therefore even more crucial that you take good care of your body.

You may never know the power of a good night's sleep in helping you revitalize your body and recover your mind. Many world changers who have ever existed are familiar with going to bed on time and waking up early. A good rest has been a precursor for living refreshed and ready to take on the new day with new strength. You can employ the same life-changing habit to conquer everyday stress.

Choose A Balanced Diet

Coming at the heels of any medical issue is mostly poor diet. You're either eating right or you're not. There's no in between with the intake of a meal that serves the body. Taking a well-nourished diet not only reduces the risk of chronic conditions but also affects your energy levels in pronounced ways.

For instance, steer clear of excessive sugars, alcohol, smoking, and other health-threatening foods. Favor water over carbonated drinks and stay hydrated as often as you can. As you grow, you may not always feel thirsty before you need water so ensure to hydrate at intervals each day. On the opposing sides, dehydration magnifies the perception of fatigue especially during a busy exercise.

Use The Hospital

If flu makes you bedridden for days rather than succumbing to a couple of pills to treat, odds are, you take the least chances at addressing physical symptoms. Your body is the house for your soul and spirit and it makes a huge difference if you would pay keen attention to visible signs.

In instances where there are no tangible signs or symptoms, it is advisable to have a medical check-up. Trips to the hospital may not be fun but they surely save you future stress and keep you afloat in your health. Maintaining synergy between you and your health practitioner would help you choose the best diet and imbibe the best medical practices.

3. Feeling Pain in Your Mind? – Do this
Unmask

We're in a world of appearances. In fact, the advent of social media bears a great margin in discouraging people from being their real self. People celebrate the picture-perfect lifestyle even if the ground they are standing on is shaking right under their feet. Sadly, many carry on with bottling up away from the media until it's too late.

Emotional stress can compound to some form of physical stress which can destabilize everyday responsibilities. The ability to get real with yourself and the courage to express what's unwell to those who will pay genuine attention is a life skill that will serve you in no small ways. Vulnerability will spearhead your healing if you allow it by sharing your deepest feelings with those who can safely accommodate it.

Share With Someone

Can I stress the importance of therapy and one-on-one once again? Through a focused session with a counselor or therapists, you can connect to the deepest parts of your innermost being and express yourself without fear of judgments. Science tells of how stress accumulates as hormones and other toxins in our body but shedding emotional tears help to ease them off and produce endorphins that act as the body's natural pain-killers.

It is okay to feel bad concerning what you can't control. So quit beating yourself up and begin to look for ways to plant yourself in environments that offer you solace and encouragement now that you need it.

Saying Goodbye to Stress

I've read various self-helps that take a typical stance on the subject of stress elimination. I put it up to you that stress isn't a one-off occurrence. While therapy sessions may initiate the process of healing, they do only so far in completely turning off the switch. The truth is, temptations will come creeping in by the time you exit your coach's office. How do you live through that?

In most cases, stress is a major trigger for anger. And the question of whether it is possible to be eaten up by stress to the point of dismissing inclinations to anger is quite common among certain parents who live on autopilot stress. Looking to suppress anger with stress is a brutal shortcut to an unhappy life and toxic home.

Fact is stress is avoidable if you involve the right strategy. Anger can be combated and subdued in the same manner. Stringing in the right steps in your day-to-day activities will rewire the default and cancerous behavior into an intentional and lively one. Right now, I can feel you're ready to take life back and retrace your steps toward living a happy and stress-free life. Let's dive in!

Take Your Life Back in Three Steps

1. Take out time to recalibrate

Taking time off from your children does not make you a terrible parent. You'll be a better parent for it. If you must get a decreased stress hormone level then relaxing is very important. For some parents, it's as easy as taking an extra five minutes to get ready in the morning. If you don't have a family member or trusted friend who can step in and give you a few hours off at a time, look for local respite programs that can help you connect with caregivers who can support you.

Don't know what to do when you're off the hook away from the intensity of caring for your children? I have titillating suggestions but first and foremost: I'll persuade you to dispose of guilt that may seek to haunt you down for excusing your child for a moment. Can I tell you that you deserve to enjoy every atom of this moment?

Now that that's all cleared up, I'll be introducing you to some getaway ideas suitable for spouses and singles alike. Go on and book an activity that pulls in your body and soul as you participate in it. The goal is to cast your mind off the rhythm of responsibility that marks your days as parents. You can try out a day trip and skywalk, water activity and river walk or enter an adventurous competition. It can even be as simple as meeting and conversing with new people.

A soothing way to spend your getaway time is to care for your body. Visit a new wine cellar and taste up what they've got in there or it could be a restaurant with new cuisines. Stop by at the gym or spa and let your body unwind.

2. Reflect

Imagine what would happen if we only slowed down our pace and stopped the ceaseless rush to success. Did I hear you mutter, "Impossible!" Viewing our world and the word 'slow' side by side is rocket science. Simply unimaginable! But what if I told you that the speed we desire is weaved into the broken fragments of a steady but sure time?

When was the last time you caught yourself mulling over something? Or sit in the sun alone with your thoughts? Or listen to your favorite song or book play aloud as you relax? Reflection is a sacrosanct stage in making quality decisions. You can go farther by keeping a journal as writing is a proven way to break down your thoughts and gather them back as gems of ideas.

Journaling is good for both men and women and you might get into the culture of keeping a strict journal or a freestyle. A strict journal is dominated by specific kinds of information. It may be a catalog of what you're grateful for or highlights of beautiful memories. You can keep an intrigue journal where you file interesting findings. It should be noted that a strict journal mainly contains positive records of events.

Alternatively, a free style journal isn't bound to certain prerequisites. Instead, they act as an open space where users can dump scraps of muses, pains, hurts, and other feelings. Also, it can include memorable letters, unforgettable findings, or any other writings you want to safeguard for a long time.

Before I set out to write my books, I remember keeping a unique journal where I poured out my heart about how frustrated I was raising a child that wouldn't listen. Then I merged contents I found interesting as I carried out my research about ADHD and Autism. A glance at that journal embodies a testimonial of how far I've come being my best as a parent. I bet that journal would never grow old even when I do and its content will remain untainted.

Meditation is highly effective in getting your mind back in the right shape. I am a terrific fan of yoga and I faithfully observe my session every morning. If you're confused about the posture, position, patterns, and direction you need for alignment, feel free to speak to a teacher. You may not necessarily observe yoga every day in order to improve your immune system and flex your muscles. However, setting apart days and times for it will prove instrumental in the long run.

3. Celebrate yourself

You can rarely get a great deed from a poor esteem. A global survey by Dove revealed that only 4% of women consider themselves beautiful. I am moved to ask what about the other 96%, what's their behavior like toward themselves and other women? Even dead-struck gorgeous women fall into the latter group.

You may say that's just a statistic pertaining to women but what I want to draw out is that even people who offer their best sometimes feel insecure and unfit. Caring for your child sure takes some balls for you not to constantly find yourself in the pit of self-doubt and second-guessing.

My friend, the reason why you may feel like you're not moving forward is because you keep raising the bar for how to raise a child well. And this underscores the fact that you're progressing and growing your abilities in being an amazing parent.

Rather than start the blame game with your spouse on who's not doing what, celebrate yourselves for how far you've come. Turn the lens on yourself for a second and sincerely appreciate the effort and grace you put into setting your child up for success despite all setbacks.

Rest assured that I will never condemn myself O'clock on anyone's planet. So, the time will never be right to engage in a war of words and deliver poisonous comebacks to yourself or spouse. Take some pride in your minute effort and move forward from there. It is more productive to have a positive self-talk than reel out condescending words.

One way to practice self-care is by showering yourself with compliments and genuinely extending it to others. Write down five tasks you're proud of yourself for completing each day at the end of the day. It might be something as small as getting to school on time or as significant as helping your child pass a new learning benchmark. Give yourself compliments in front of your kids as well.

Balancing Parental Responsibilities

True, in a society where everyone aspires to reach their goals, many parents find it hard to achieve balance, particularly when it comes to juggling the demands of raising a kid with special needs and taking care of themselves. For this reason, before I end this chapter, I felt compelled to emphasize this. When it comes to handling the pressure of your responsibilities as a parent, your ability to maintain equilibrium will determine whether you get easily overwhelmed or remain motionless. I'll outline some doable actions you can take to strike this balance in the ensuing paragraphs.

1. Make Time Management A Priority

You might be shocked to hear that not just your child with ADHD has to learn time management skills, but you too. Plan ahead for everything you need to do and give each task a specific amount of time. Schedule time for your self-care in the same way that you do for your assignment. This will assist you in avoiding pointless activities.

2. Assign And Look for Assistance

Who said you have to work alone on this? When help is needed, ask for it. Involve your family and other experts. In the previous chapter of this book, I discussed working with specialists to parent your child who has special needs.

Working together will benefit you in many ways, one of which is that it will allow you to take time for yourself.

3. Set Realistic Goals

It is imperative that one sets realistic goals. This cannot be overstated. Nothing is more frustrating than having a goal that is not reached. Set SMART goals.

When raising a child with special needs, do you find that you become quickly agitated? Or you've made multiple attempts to manage your anger. You should read the following chapter. I'm going to walk you through some doable strategies for controlling your rage.

The next chapter will offer you pearls of knowledge to assist you in managing anger issues with your neurodiverse child.

TAKE HOME:

- Your self-care is important if you must parent your special-needs child effectively.

- Your Ability to balance your parental responsibilities and your self-care is what will determine how you will handle the difficulties that may arise as you parent your child.

- Nothing is more frustrating than having a goal that is not reached. Set Realistic goals.

CHAPTER FIVE

PRACTICAL TIPS FOR ANGER MANAGEMENT

"Anger is like a storm rising up from the bottom of your consciousness. When you feel it coming, turn your focus to your breath."

-Thich Nhat Hanh

In the previous chapter, you got insights into the privileges of collaborating with professionals and therapists. Also, the chapter exposed you to individualized parenting strategies for children with ADHD and Autism. Here, you are going to familiarize yourself with how to manage your anger when dealing with a neurodiverse child.

Being a parent is a tough gig; there's no doubt about that. There will be moments that are beautiful lifelong memories. Others will try your patience and leave you wondering if it's all worth it. It's not a question of if, but when you as a parent will lose your temper with your child.

Of course, kids don't know any better and they will push you to the edge. The danger is when your anger spills over onto your child, crushing their self-esteem, hurting their feelings, or making them feel unwanted. Understanding how your anger can change your child's environment for the worse, and how it can impact their growth is key in helping you curtail it. Nobody wants an unhappy child, and you owe it to your children to prevent their unhappiness. Managing anger is a huge component of raising a happy, healthy, and emotionally intelligent child.

Anger is a natural and healthy emotion, serving as the counterpart to positive emotions like joy and happiness. Most individuals can express anger in a constructive manner without it turning into a negative experience or harming others. It is an evolutionary response deeply connected to our need for survival. When confronted with anger, one may respond by either confronting the source (fight), distancing oneself from it (flight), or feeling immobilized by fury (freeze). Experiencing anger on a regular basis is normal and can be a motivating force, compelling individuals to take action and address issues. Anger, far from being a negative force, is an essential and constructive emotion.

The Story of Amelia

Amelia felt her pulse quicken as she entered the therapy room, her mind a whirlwind of emotions. Her sessions with Dr. Thompson had been a lifeline, guiding her through the maze of emotions that came with parenting an autistic child.

One sunny afternoon, as she sat with her son, Nathan, the familiar triggers began to surface like bubbles on simmering water. His frustration was palpable, yet Amelia felt a newfound calmness wash over her. Remembering Dr. Thompson's advice, she took a deep breath, allowing the air to fill her lungs slowly, and then released it, willing the tension to dissipate.

Nathan's agitation grew, echoing her own internal struggle. But this time, Amelia was different. She no longer felt consumed by anger but instead viewed the situation through a clearer lens. With each inhale and exhale, she centered herself, recognizing that Nathan's actions were a reflection of his own frustrations, not a personal attack.

She remembered the therapist's words: "Respond, don't react." Taking this mantra to heart, she chose her words carefully, speaking in a soothing tone. She offered a comforting touch, guiding Nathan through his emotions.

In those moments of deep breathing and deliberate actions, Amelia found herself connected to her child in a profound way. She felt the tension ebb away, replaced by a sense of understanding and empathy.

As the afternoon unfolded, Nathan's agitation gradually subsided. Amelia noticed a remarkable change in herself – a newfound sense of maturity and resilience. She realized that practicing these exercises wasn't just for her benefit but also for creating a more harmonious environment for Nathan.

With each passing day, Amelia continued to integrate these techniques into her routine. Deep breathing became her anchor, guiding her through the turbulent waters of parenting an autistic child. She discovered that in moments of frustration, the power of pausing, breathing, and responding mindfully transformed not only her reactions but also her relationship with Nathan.

Deep Breathing

Use deep breathing to invoke a sense of peace and calm and to counteract rising tension. Concentrate on the breath going in and out of the lungs to take the focus off the source of the anger. It is important to take deep breaths rather than breathing shallowly from the chest, as that technique is not as effective. One way to ensure this happens is to use a specific deep breathing technique:

- Close the mouth and inhale breath through the nose for approximately 4 seconds

- Hold for 7 seconds

- Release the air through the mouth for 8 seconds. This has a tranquilizing effect on the nervous system and will alleviate anger.

Mindfulness Techniques

Using mindfulness to feel your anger is one way you can connect with your emotions, process them, and help yourself feel more relaxed. Here are a few steps to help in your mindfulness.

1. **Mindful Meditation**: Practice mindfulness meditation, focusing on the present moment without judgment. It helps in creating a sense of calm and detachment from emotions.

2. **Visualize what made you angry**: You can think about an incident that triggered your anger. You may want to picture all the details until you can feel your anger rising.

3. **Take a Pause**: When feeling angry, take a moment before responding. This pause allows you to choose a more thoughtful response rather than reacting impulsively.

4. **Mindful Walking or Movement**: Engage in mindful walking or movement exercises. Pay attention to each

step or movement, focusing on the sensations and the environment around you.

5. **Gratitude Practice**: Cultivate gratitude by focusing on positive aspects of your life. This can help shift your perspective and reduce feelings of anger.

6. **Progressive Muscle Relaxation**: Practice muscle relaxation techniques by tensing and then relaxing different muscle groups. This can help release physical tension and promote relaxation.

An Emily Story

Emily's days were often a whirlwind of activity and emotions. Her son, Alex, a vibrant and creative young boy with autism, brought joy but also moments of intense challenge. One evening, as she juggled dinner preparations and Alex's need for attention, frustration bubbled up within her. Recognizing the familiar signs of escalating tension, Emily excused herself gently from the bustling kitchen. She left Alex engaged in his favorite activity, and in her bedroom, she closed the door, seeking a moment of respite.

Sitting on the edge of the bed, Emily focused on her breathing. Inhale, exhale – the rhythmic pattern became her anchor in the sea of emotions. She acknowledged the mounting frustration and the need for a moment to collect her thoughts.

In her mind's eye, Emily visualized a serene garden she had once visited, a peaceful place where she found solace. The mental imagery transported her momentarily from the chaos of the household, providing a brief reprieve.

As she continued to breathe deeply, a sense of calmness washed over her. The initial surge of frustration began to subside. Emily took a few more moments, allowing herself the space to reset and gain perspective.

Returning to the living room, Emily found Alex engrossed in his toys. Instead of reacting with impatience or tension, she approached him with a softer demeanor. She initiated a calm and positive interaction, redirecting the energy of the moment.

In the subsequent days, Emily made it a practice to utilize these time-out moments. Whether it was a brief pause or a step away from a challenging situation, these intentional breaks became a vital tool in managing her emotions. She discovered that by taking a moment to breathe and reset, she could respond more calmly and effectively to Alex's needs, fostering a more peaceful environment for both of them.

If you can control your feelings, you can get your child and home under control. Today, unsatisfied parents pout mouths and frown faces at misunderstanding and impatience that have eaten deeply into the fabric of their home. They worry about the strain that anger's unpredictability has caused them and shed secret tears.

While I can't deny that life can be a rollercoaster of events leaving us without a moment's notice to prepare, what I can also argue is that we can divorce worry by doing a single thing. That is, get good at putting yourself under control. You see, worry arises when we make plans to control circumstances that are beyond our sphere of influence. That's an effortless way to prepare for premium frustration.

For instance, an attempt to control your ADHD or Autistic child is a fruitless goal. But if you would only turn around and demand peace from yourself as a parent in your home, it's just a matter of time when your example will spread over every member of your household like a thick cozy blanket.

Time Out Strategies for Parents to Reduce Anger

Time outs are good for kids as well as adults. I mean adults who care to move from a grumpy state to a more altruistic one. Recall how you can put a toy in time out if your child is fighting with another child over the toy or sending two siblings entangled in ceaseless bouts of fighting in immediate time-out. It works well for parents too.

The following time-out steps will serve its purpose when you apply it as remedy to help reduce anger:

1. *Have a mix of time-ins and time-outs:* Positive reinforcement is common to time-ins. It's when you

invest the time in praising, looking after, and spoiling yourself with attention. You can translate it as your self-awareness period. Contrastingly, time out is when you remove yourself from the umbrella of this devout time-usage and you just let life whirl by.

A good dose of time-ins will imprint on your life in capital ways that you'll spend little time in time-outs. At the same time, a dash of time-out here and there will put you in a state to examine the dividends of operating in an amazing time-in when you're ready.

2. *Make it immediate, consistent, and brief:* One liberty you have as a parent is you get to call the shots. And having to lead yourself into starting and finishing a task should reflect that you're in charge of yourself. Time-outs are effective when used as a tool of change rather than a luxury of leisure.

If you catch yourself caught in a heated argument with your child, take a time-out immediately. You don't have to wait until you see it through or win the argument. Take a backward step into the confines of a time-out and do it on time.

3. ***Change your mind set about time-outs:*** Viewing time-outs as a relapse rather than a recovery will empower you to manifest time-in-worthy behaviors in the long run. When you arrange time-outs sessions into a stretch of boring disengagements, you might have a change of heart about constantly falling behind on the good deeds.

   Make time-outs as uninteresting as possible and odds are you would think twice in the ways you express your feelings so as to avoid putting yourself to the unceremonious test of time-outs.

Consistency is key to the effectiveness of these strategies and regular reflection on their impact allows you to refine and tailor these practices to fit different unique situations. When you start having no need for time-outs, it might just be a pointer that you're getting your feelings together. So, keep on keeping on!

TAKE HOME:

- Anger is a natural and healthy emotion, serving as the counterpart to positive emotions like joy and happiness

- Being mindful of one's emotions allows parents to acknowledge and understand their anger without judgment.

- Incorporating deep breathing exercises provides a practical and immediate way to calm the nervous system and release physical tension.

- Implementing intentional breaks, or time-outs, enables parents to step back, collect their thoughts, and regain composure before responding to challenging situations.

CONCLUSION

Peace has never been a bad deal for anyone who offers it. And for parents of ADHD and Autistic parents, negotiating peace isn't enough: you have to settle for peace beyond word of mouth. The kind of peace that will put the ambiance of your home under control has to be worked out in your actions and in-actions.

No doubt, the previous pages have constituted a knowledge-bank you can draw from to tackle the tension you feel with your neurodiverse child hands-on. Through the insights and experiments laden with relevant research work, this book has proven to be an adequate resource with an exceptional assistance in helping you dislodge anger from your parent-child and parent-parent relationships.

In Chapter 1, you understood why your ADHD or Autistic child is different and why you need to pay extra attention to your child because of that. This chapter presented you with possible influences that your child's uniqueness might have on your parenting dynamic. It gave a prelude to how your parenting styles may affect your child which is later discussed in full in Chapter 3.

Chapter 2 connected the subtle dots between parenting, stress, and anger. Through my story as a mother of autistic child coupled with the stories of some parents with neurodiverse children, you got inside information on the various ways that stress and anger can materialize in a parent's life. The chapter opened your eyes to the reality of these struggles and suggested a coping mechanism you can apply a time a day.

We all come to our wits end as parents and must look outside to seek help that will suffice for the troubles ravaging our home. Here, Chapter 3 offered instances for obtaining professional help from therapists and consultants. It detailed what you need to do while preparing to get one and how to maximize its impact once it is underway. Speaking to a professional can turn out as the solution you desperately need and this chapter exposes you to the intricacies.

Chapter 4 discussed self-care as a tool for finding inner peace in order to maintain external quiet. It offers a plethora of ways to tune-in to your feelings, record your pain, heal through special practices, and take out stress altogether. It offers you practical guidelines on how to achieve balance as you disseminate your parental responsibilities and unveils the treasures of living above emotional turmoil.

Chapter 5 laid out steps for every parent interested in winning the war over. Although the chapter has been named Practical Skills for Anger Management, its content runs deeper in exposing the techniques and practices necessary to achieve consistent changes. By examining the layers of stories of ADHD and Autistic children whose parents had tough times handling, you will be inspired by how these parents looked for the missing link and steadily bridged the gap that hindered the flow of communication.

No two homes are the same. Yet, by considering the ebbs and flows and patterns of parents with similar neurodiverse backgrounds, it is possible to create a rhythm that will hold your own family in unity and put negativity out.

Your Free Gift

As a way of saying thanks for your purchase, I'm offering this book ***BABY SAFETY TIPS*** for **FREE** to my readers.

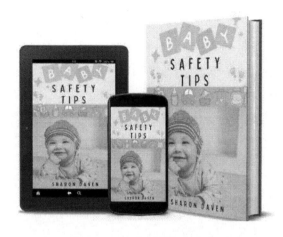

To get instant access **SCAN THE QR CODE:**

Inside this book, you will discover:

- 12-Must have products that will keep your child safe around the home

- Traveling with a baby checklist.

- How to reduce the risk of poisoning in your household.

- Toy Safety Tips.

- Safe bedding practices for infants

If you want to know how to keep your baby safe, make sure to grab this **FREE** book now.

Authors Note

Dear Reader,

I hope you enjoyed reading my book as much as I enjoyed writing it. Your feedback means the world to me, and I'd be incredibly grateful if you could take a moment to *leave a review.*

The review will not only brighten my day but also help other potential readers discover the book.

So, please, share your thoughts, insights and feelings about this book. Thank you for your support.

Warmest wishes,

Sharon Daven

REFERENCES

1. Balancing the Demands of Parenthood and Self-Care. https://www.sunshinecitycounseling.com/blog/balancing-parenthood-and-self-care?format=amp

2. Baumrind, D. (2005). Patterns of parental authority and adolescent autonomy. New Directions for Child and Adolescent Development, 108, 61–69.

3. Brandt, A. (2014). Mindful anger: a pathway to emotional freedom. Noroton Professional Books.

4. Cosmopolitan. (2013). Most women don't feel beautiful. https://www.cosmopolitan.com/style-beauty/beauty/news/a11997/most-women-dont-think-theyre-beautiful/

5. Deater-Deckard, K. (2008). Parenting stress. Yale University Press.

6. Eastridge, D. (2013). Anger management and coping skills. Learning Services Neuro.

7. Kleiven GS, et al. (2020). Opening up: Clients' inner struggles in the initial phase of therapy. https://www.frontiersin.org/articles/10.3389/fpsyg.2020.591146/full

8. Loewenstein, G. (1996). Out of control: Visceral influences on behavior. Organizational behavior and human decision processes, 65(3), 272-292.

9. Malcom, S. (2022). Anger management for parents: how to successfully deal with emotions & raise happy and confident kids.

10. Neurodiversity at work: a biopsychosocial model and the impact on working adults - PMC https://www.ncbi.nlm.nih.gov/pmc/articles/PMC773203 3/#bib1title

11. Neurodiversity - NCI https://dceg.cancer.gov/about/diversity-inclusion/inclusivity-minute/2022/neurodiversity

12. Parenting styles: An evidence-based, cross-cultural guide https://parentingscience.com/parenting-styles/

13. Self-Care for Parents of Kids with Behavioral Challenges. https://www.brainbalancecenters.com/blog/self-care-behavioral-challenges

14. Talking therapies. (n.d.). https://www.rethink.org/advice-and-information/living-with-mental-illness/treatment-and-support/talking-therapies/

15. The Benefits of Support Groups | Arizona Addiction Recovery Center. https://arizonaaddictioncenter.org/the-benefits-of-support-groups/

16. Therapy and Neurodivergence – Newglade Counselling – Neurodivergent Services.

https://newgladecounselling.co.uk/2021/10/25/therapy-and-neurodivergence/

17. Wing, L. (2013). Autistic children: a guide for parents & professionals. Routledge.

18. https://www.parenthelp.org.nz/parenting-style/

Made in the USA
Las Vegas, NV
04 November 2024

cd819b0f-8c74-4b5c-955a-b68706eac896R01